The Orthopaedic Intern Pocket Survival Guide

Derek H. Ochiai, MD

Other titles from International Medical Publishing:

The Intern Pocket Survival Guide
The CCU Intern Pocket Survival Guide
The Surgical Intern Pocket Survival Guide
The ICC Intern Pocket Survival Guide
The Oncology Intern Pocket Survival Guide

The EKG Pocket Survival Guide
The ACLS Pocket Survival Guide

Published by International Medical Publishing, Inc.
PO Box 479
McLean, VA 22101
800-530-3142
fax: 703-734-8987

ISBN 1-58808-080-3

Printed in U.S.A.

To Emmeline and Whitman

Contents

Introduction

"The truth of the matter is that you always know the right thing to do. The hard part is doing it."
—General H. Norman Schwarzkopf, 1991.

Orthopaedic surgery, in many cases, takes healthy patients and tries to decrease pain and increase function. A good outcome is expected; a bad outcome is laid at the feet of the attending. Since these patients for the most part do not need surgery to save their lives, it is especially important to avoid complications. All orthopaedic patients must receive every aspect of standard preoperative and postoperative care. Further, attendings need to be kept apprised of all unexpected patient developments.

Gaining the respects of peers and medical staff comes from the application of the golden rule: treat others as you would have them treat you. Show respect towards nurses, staff, and medical students by remembering and using their names.

Success as a new orthopaedic surgery resident requires diligence, hard work, and conscientiousness. Be completely truthful. It is easy to say a lab was checked when it wasn't, but that will be the time the attending decides to check it out. Get into the OR as much as possible. This is valuable "face time" with the attendings that will help later on, and lead to operating time.

The information in this book is not meant to be comprehensive. Please refer to the reading list found in the back of the book.

NB: Please consult with your resident before trying anything new.

The Laws of Internship

1. Listen when nature calls

2. Make time for meals

3. Sleep whenever possible

4. Call spouse or significant other when on call

Pre-Op – Daily Organization

"Just because I'm paranoid doesn't mean they're not out to get me."

How to Organize a Typical Day.

Pre-Preround: Get the list for the patients on your service. Make sure to check with the person on call from the night before for any patients that may not be on your list and a heads up for any problems.

Preround: Tmax, VSS, drain outputs, neurovascular exam of extremity, full neuro exam on spine patients

Check labs and consult notes from the other services.

Notes done before rounds.

Rounds: Present patients concisely—name, age, diagnosis/procedure, post op day, any unusual course (DVT, infection).

Mention: Vitals, pertinent exam findings and labs, meds started in house (anti-coagulation, antibiotics).

Find out plans for removing drains, weightbearing, PT, and discharge.

Write down all of the plans at the time they are discussed. Do not rely on memory!

Post rounds:

1. Write orders for each patient, especially labs, PT, X-ray. In a busy hospital, if some orders are not received in the morning, it won't get done or will be done late.
2. Call OR scheduling desk to add on patients.
3. Discharge patients. It helps to have a good relationship with the discharge planner.
4. Check labs. Correct any electrolyte abnormalities and adjust anti-coagulation. Drop an addendum in the chart.
5. Call consults. The earlier they are called, the earlier you get an answer.
6. Hustle to the OR if needed. If not, get some food.
7. Do everything your senior told you to do.

Pre-Op – Daily Organization (continued)

Afternoon Rounds: Alert team to any problems that crept up during the day (labs, temp, falls, problems with PT, D/C problems).

8. End of day checklist for every patient
   –AM labs, tests for tomorrow
   –Pre-op note for tomorrow's surgery patients
   –Post-op check for today's surgery patients
9. Gather list for sign out. Write on a sheet what needs to be done for each patient. Include add-on cases for that evening, important labs to check, critical patients.

NOW GO HOME. Take a little time to read about cases you might be doing the next day, or a topic for conference.

Pre-Op – Miscellaneous Organization

"I've had good days, and bad days, and going half mad days"—Jimmy Buffett

–Let your resident know early about any complications or problems with patients. Nobody is going to pat you on the back for managing a problem correctly without at least informing your senior, but everyone will kick your butt for incorrectly managing a problem without informing your senior

–Intervene by day, rest by night. Pull drains, adjust meds, check X-rays and labs early so that if you need help, it's available.

–It is safer to check a patient out yourself and write a note rather than trust a description over the phone.

–If it's truly important, delegate the task to yourself.

–Consult early, consult often. This will differ by institution. In general, Ortho is not expected to manage alone any serious medical condition.

–Discharge planning begins on the day of admission.

–Medical students deserve education time from you. Take care of your students and you'll find the medical students more helpful to you in return.

Admission Checklist

"Every patient is a pre-op for something."
As soon as you learn about the patient, ask for old charts. This can save you a lot of legwork.

1. Admission H&P
2. Pre-op labs, Type and Screen, EKG, X-rays, medical clearance
3. Consent for surgery signed, including the correct side (right or left)
4. Write pre-op note when all labs, clearance in place

Pre-Op – Admission H&P

"When I see lengthy notes from the surgical housestaff, I know they don't have enough to do."—West Coast, General Surgery Program Director

You are not a medical student anymore. Don't fill an H&P with useless junk. An orthopaedic H&P can be completed in two pages or less.

History
- CC
- HPI
- PMH
- PSH
- Meds
- Allergies
- FH
- SH (smoking, ETOH, IVDA)

Physical Exam
- Vitals, including temp, pulse ox
- Neck: Lymphadenopathy, JVD, supple
- Heart: obvious murmurs, arthymias
- Lungs: Clear BS B/L
- Ab: soft, non-tender, non-distended, normoactive bowel sounds
- Extremity: Moves all four extremities, check ROM of all joints, document any neurovascular abnormalities pre-op (ie. Wrist drop, no dorsalis pedis pulse)

Labs, U/A
CXR, extremity X-ray
EKG

A/P It's OK to be general here. The choice of repair belongs to the attending.

Spinal Cord Injuries-special consideration given to P.E. because change in exam can be a clue to a good prognosis or devastating complication! Individual motor and sensory strength must be known for each level (see pages 68–70). Every spinal cord injury patient gets a rectal exam for tone, perianal sensation and bulbocavernosus reflex. Every spine injury patient should be carefully moved off the backboard (while maintaining spine precautions) to decrease risk of decubitus ulcers.

Pre-Op – Admission EKG

Run any abnormalities by your resident to see if a cardiology consult is indicated.

1. Get an old EKG for comparison.

2. Systematic Examination:
   –Rhythm
   –Rate
   –Intervals
      PR <.21 seconds
      QRS <.12
      Qt˚
   –Axis – 3 to +120˚
   –then PQRST…
      P wave morphology
      Q waves
      R wave progression
      ST – segments – quantify elevation or depression
      T waves

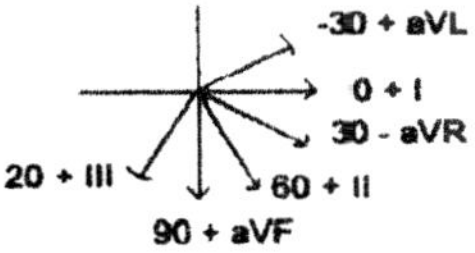

Rate:
Each of the little boxes is 0.04 sec and 5 boxes 0.2 sec.
Heart rate: one beat per big box =300bpm, 2=150, 3+100, 4=75 5=60, and 6=50.

ST Segments:
Ischemia – depression.
Infarction – elevation.
(reciprocal changes.)

Distribution of Infarction:
Anterior – precordial (V_2-V_8)
Inferior – II, III, aVF.
Lateral – I, aVL, V_5 V_8
Posterior – reciprocal, large R in V_1 – V_2 ST depression in V_1-V_2

Take advantage of the medical residents for looking at EKGs. If there is any question, get a formal reading (this may be required in some institutions).

Pre-Op – Admission CXR

"If I wanted the X-ray report tomorrow, I would have ordered it tomorrow."

If an incompletely evaluated trauma patient has found his way onto your service, make sure your resident is aware of your concerns and have a low threshold for consulting the trauma or ICU services.

Read your own films in a systematic fashion. Always start with the name and date. Get the radiologist to review them with you whenever possible.

CXR:

- Name, date, technique, rotation.
- Placement of all lines and tubes – NG tube should be in stomach, end of central line, end of endrotracheal tube, location of PA catheter.
- Bones, e.g. shoulder, rib, fx, spine. Look for subcutaneous emphysema.
- Mediastinum:
    - Aortic knob widened?
    - Hilum.
    - Cardiac silhouette.

Lung fields:

- Pneumothorax? pneumomediastinum?
- Pneumoperitoneum?
- Bases, effusion (compare with lateral).
- Cardiac borders, vessels.
- Apices. capping?
- Left vs. right – lobar, interstitial, nodules.

Kerley As head to the apex.
Kerley Bs are short lines laterally.

Look at the lateral – identify both diaphragms.

In ruling out a pneumothorax, make sure the film was upright. Always use a hot light. Order a second film if there are any persistent concerns.

Pre-Op – Orthopaedic X-rays

Always look at your own films. The attending radiologist is a great resource, but in the middle of the night, you could be getting a wet read from someone with less training than you.

Spine X-rays

C-spine-Lateral X-ray will be diagnostic on a majority of C-spine injuries. Make sure that you can visualize the entire C-spine from atlas to top of T1. Otherwise, redo the film, pulling down on the patient's arms to get the shoulders out of the way or get a swimmer's view. Anterior vertebral, posterior vertebral, and spinolaminar lines should all be smooth. Be aware of pseudosubluxation of C2-3 in young children (normal). 5 views are a complete series. If in doubt, call senior and consider CT scan.

TLS spine-Lateral should show a normal thoracic kyphosis and lumbar lordosis. Lateral is best for seeing compression fractures, spondylolisthesis. A/P is good for confirming burst fracture (by interpedicular widening) or subluxation in coronal plane. Obliques are good for showing spondylolysis (collar on the Scottie dog).

Extremity X-rays in general—Get at least two views at 90 degrees to each other for each fracture. For long bone fractures, x-rays must include the joint above and below site of fracture (ie femur fractures have 10% incidence of associated hip fractures). If a fracture is seen on x-ray that you are not sure of, look it up to see if additional views are necessary. These other views are much easier to get in the ER than after the patient is admitted and on the floor. If you see a patient with a grossly displaced fracture or dislocation, check vascular status of the limb. If the skin is blanched, pulses diminished, or loss of motor/sensory, call senior and reduce the fracture before getting X-rays.

Shoulder X-rays

An orthopaedic trauma series include A/P, lateral, and AXILLARY view. Posterior dislocations are easy to miss without axillary view. The X-ray techs will universally tell you that they can't get it because they don't want to move the patient's shoulder. Position the patient yourself, abducting the arm about 35 degrees. Patients can tolerate this, especially if you are holding their arm.

Hip X-rays

With suspected hip fractures, include an A/P pelvis so you can compare sides and also catch any associated pelvic injury

Pre-Op – Admission Orders

Admit to Ortho Attending _____ Resident _____ Intern ______

Dx:

Condition

Vitals (q6hrs on routine floor, q1 in ICU), neurovascular checks for extremity in jeopardy

Activities: Encourage incentive spirometry, OOB, weightbearing restrictions

Allergies: specific or NKDA

Nursing strict I/O's (including drains)

- Ted's hose +/- SCD's
- Drains to gravity/suction/reinfusion protocol
- Decubitus precautions

Diet: Regular, NPO after midnight for presurgical patients

IVF: Heplock IV, give D51/2 NS at 100 cc/hr if NPO for surgery

Meds: Resume all meds as appropriate

- If patient is on cardiac, pulmonary meds, can usually take with sips of water if NPO.
- Hold insulin/diabetic meds if patient NPO and cover with sliding scale of regular insulin (may have medical consult to help manage diabetes).
- Anti-coagulation if appropriate (Warfarin, low molecular weight heparin)

Labs: CBC, PT, PTT, Chem 8, U/A, C&S

X-rays as appropriate

PT/OT consults

Social Services

Discharge planning

Be aware of comorbidities such as renal disease or CHF. Refer any questions to your senior. Don't rely on consultants to write orders unless they specifically say they will write them. Consultants will only write orders that relate to them, so you still have to write admission orders!

Call the patient's medical attending and let them know the patient is in-house.

Pre-Op Note

The pre-op note is essentially a checklist written into the progress notes confirming that all of the data has been gathered and the patient is ready for surgery.

Pt is pre-op for ______________(date)
CBC (also look at platelets)
PT/PTT
Medical clearance if necessary
T&S or T&C 2 units (perhaps more if major pelvic/acetabular/ tumor surgery)
Consent on the chart
Pre-op orders written

PRE-OP Orders

Frequently these are included in the admission orders:

NPO after MN
IVF's
Antibiotics (usually Ancef unless allergic) to go with patient to OR.

Pre-Op Consent

"Our therapeutic efforts also have special significance to him. How will this operation affect his life? Does it carry an immediate threat to life itself? Is he to suffer more pain and then be free from it?"—Austen Riggs, MD, 1928

"We may not be able to make you better, but we can surely make you different."—Anonymous surgeon

A valid consent performs several tasks:

1. Provides warning-risks of the procedure
2. Informs patient-cognizant of the planned procedure and the alternatives
3. Grants permission to perform the procedure

Obtaining consent for a procedure or operation is a vital step for both you and the patient. Without consent, surgery may be battery.

Is the patient capable of providing consent? Social workers can often help locate the surrogate decision-maker for the patient.

Check with senior or attending regarding how the consent is to read. The consent should include all actual planned procedures as well as potential procedures. For example, a consent for surgery for a hip fracture could read "Percutaneous pinning right hip, possible ORIF, possible hemiarthroplasti." The goal is to translate into English the mechanics of the procedure and its possible risks. For example, for the hip fracture: "We will put you on a special x-ray table and look at the fracture. If we feel it can be fixed through small poke holes and pins, we will do that. Sometimes a larger incision needs to be made to get the bone in good alignment. And sometimes, we find the break is too bad to be put back together, and we need to replace the ball of your hip, giving you half a total hip replacement." Do not go into details about what type of implant will be put in unless you know specifically from the attending.

Pre-Op Consent (continued)

In addition to procedure-specific complications, include the general complications, which include, but are not limited to, the risks of anesthesia, bleeding, the need for transfusion, and infection. If the patient is at a significant risk for a complicated postoperative course due to co-morbidities (i.e. diabetes for infection and wound dehiscence) this needs to be communicated to the patient and documented in the consent.

Frequently, a separate form is required for possible blood transfusions. If the patient does not want a blood transfusion, discuss this with your senior. Many times, patients with a strong aversion to blood transfusions will consent to possible transfusion if it is stated clearly "We will do everything possible to avoid giving you blood. However, sometimes, even with these efforts, it is necessary to give you blood to save your life."

Get the consent early in the day on the day prior to surgery. Do not leave consents for the sign-out. Always sign the consent. Witnesses are required, and they should also sign the consent. A note should be placed in the chart indicating the procedure was discussed with the patient, and that the patient understands the risks and the potential benefits of the procedure and consents to surgery.

Pre-Op Studies

Certain tests and procedures are required of all patients prior to undergoing elective or routine procedures. The exact tests will depend upon the surgery, type of anesthesia, co-morbidities, patient condition, and local idiosyncrasies.

CBC
PT/PTT
U/A, C&S
Beta-HCG (females, may be done in ER)
EKG, CXR (over 40, any risk factors)
T&S, T&C 2-6 units (procedure dependent)
Any other test that consultants deem necessary.

Pre-Op Antibiotics

"The heart is a necessary organ to pump the Ancef around."—Anonymous Orthopaedic Surgeon

For orthopaedic procedures, Ancef is normally the drug of choice. Don't reflexively order it without first thinking of complicating factors.

Elective procedure	Ancef 1 gm IV Clindamycin 600 mg IV or Vancomycin 1 gm IV (if allergic)
Open fractures	Type I/II-Ancef 1gm IV q8 hr for 3 days Type III-Ancef plus Gentamycin 1.5 mg/kg q 8 hrs for 5 days Type III with barnyard, lake or stream contamination-add Penicillin 4 million units q6hrs for clostridium prophylaxis (see Open Fractures for classification, page 66)

Antibiotics are given just prior to the case in the OR or in the ER. Many times, patients will say they are allergic to penicillin. Cephalosporin cross-reaction is of much greater concern if the penicillin reaction was anaphylaxis.

Operative Dictation

Plan to dictate any case where you play a significant role. Clarify specimens, findings, and all diagnoses before dictating. Anesthesia will provide an estimate on fluids in and out, as well as blood loss.

This is Dr. ______________ dictating operative note on

Patient name
Medical record number
Date of surgery
Pre-op diagnosis
Post-op diagnosis
Procedure
Attending: ______________
Assistants: ______________
Anesthesia: (General, epidural, spinal, regional block, local)
EBL
IVF
Drains
Complications
Disposition (i.e. to PACU in stable condition)

Indications for surgery (i.e. 65 year old with significant right knee osteoarthritis. He has failed conservative management. He was seen by Dr. ______________ in the office and felt to be an appropriate candidate for right total knee replacement. Informed consent was obtained prior to surgery.)

Description of Operative Procedures/Findings

1. Position
2. Draping
3. Incision and approach
4. Describe pathology
5. Therapeutic intervention
6. Location of drains
7. Type of closure

This is the end of dictation on patient name, medical record number by Dr. ______________. Thank you.

If your hospital dictation system gives a confirmation number after the dictation, write it down in the chart.

Intertrochanteric Hip Fracture ORIF Dictation

The following dictations are provided as sample reports. The choice of implants and suture materials is surgeon/institution specific.

The patient was taken to the operating room and placed under general anesthesia. 1 gm of Ancef was given for infection prophylaxis. The patient was then transferred to the fracture table. The right hip was secured to the traction boot, and the left leg was placed in the semi-lithotomy position. C-arm X-ray was used to visualize the fracture in both the A/P and lateral projections. Incremental traction and internal rotation was applied until an adequate reduction was obtained. The hip was then prepped with alcohol and iodine and a standard shower curtain drape was applied.

An approximately 10 cm lateral incision was made on the right leg starting at the level of the greater trochanter and extending distally. Once through the skin and subcutaneous tissue, any bleeders were cauterized with the Bovie. The fascia of the iliotibial band was visualized. A deep knife was used to cut the IT band longitudinally in line with its fibers. The fascia of the vastus lateralis was then visualized. The fascia was cut longitudinally, and a Key elevator was used to bluntly dissect through the muscle and expose the femur, taking care to cauterize any feeding vessels encountered. The fracture was visualized.

At this point, a guide pin was inserted using the 135 degree drill guide into the femoral head starting laterally at the level of the lesser trochanter. The guide pin was visualized in both the A/P and lateral planes entering the head, and the position was in the center of the head. The pin was advanced until it was 5 mm from the subchondral bone. The depth gauge was used and measured 96 mm. The triple reamer calibrated to 95 mm, and then reamed over the guide pin. We elected to use a 95 mm lag screw and a four hole 135 degree side plate. The plate/screw construct was screwed in over the guide pin, and the candlestick impactor was used to impact the plate to the femur. Care was taken to have the side plate flush with the bone. A Verbrugge was used to secure the plate Each hole was separately drilled, tapped, and secured with cortical screws ranging from 34-38 mm. At this point, the traction was gently reduced, and a compression screw was used to compress the fracture and left in place.

The wound was then thoroughly irrigated with normal saline, and closure was begun. The fascia overlying the vastus lateralis was closed with a running 0-Vicryl. A hemovac drain was then placed so the the trocar pierced the anterior portion of the IT band, exiting the skin anterior and distal to the incision. The IT band was closed with number 1 Vicryl figure of eight sutures. The subcutaneous tissue was closed with 2-0 Vicryl, and staples were used to close the skin. A sterile dressing was applied, and the patient went to PACU in stable condition.

Hemi-arthroplasty for Femoral Neck Fracture Dictation

The patient was brought to the operating room suite and placed under general anesthesia. 1 gm of Ancef was given for infection prophylaxis. The patient was then placed in the lateral decubitus position, left side up. Padded bolsters were used to secure the patient. An axillary roll was placed under the right axilla. The leg was prepped with alcohol and betadine to below the knee. The hip was sterilely draped. An approximately 15 cm incision was used, centered on the greater trochanter, extending laterally down the femur and gently curved posteriorly proximally. A standard posterior approach was utilized. Once through the skin and subcutaneous tissue, a Bovie cautery device was used on the superficial bleeders. The tensor fascia latae was incised with a deep knife, and the gluteus maximus was bluntly split inline with its fibers proximally. At this point, a Charnley retractor was utilized. The femur was gently internally rotated, putting the short external rotators on stretch. The piriformis was visualized, tagged with a suture, then released. The short external rotators were then released at their insertion on the femur and reflected laterally to protect the sciatic nerve. The sciatic nerve was palpated with a finger to ensure that it was away from the operative site. The capsule had been torn from the fracture, and the rest of the capsule was released, exposing the fracture and the head.

A bone hook was used to clear the shaft from the head, and a corkscrew was used to remove the head in one piece. The head measured to 48 mm. The acetabulum was irrigated to clear any remaining bone fragments. A 48 sizer was found to have a good fit. At this point, a femoral neck retractor was used to elevate the shaft. A cookie cutter was used first with appropriate anteversion, and then sequential broaches were introduced up to a size 13. A cement restrictor was placed distally and the shaft was thoroughly irrigated and cleaned. A size 12 stem was cemented in place, using a pressurizer. Once the stem was set in place, a 48 mm trial head was used. The hip was stable in position of sleep, and stable at 90 degrees of flexion and 60 degrees of internal rotation. The permanent femoral head was impacted onto the Morse taper of the stem and the hip was reduced.

The wound was thoroughly irrigated and closure was begun. The remaining capsule was closed with number 1 Vicryl. A hemovac drain was placed, exiting anterior and distal to the wound. The piriformis was re-approximated with number 1 Vicryl. The fascia latae was closed with number 1 Vicryl interrupted figure of eights, and the gluteus fascia was closed with running number 1 Vicryl. The deep subcutaneous tissue was closed with 0-Vicryl, the superficial subcutaneous tissue was closed with 2-0 Vicryl, and staples were used to close the skin. A sterile dressing was applied and the patient went to PACU in stable condition.

Ankle Fracture ORIF Dictation

The patient was brought to the operating room. Spinal anesthesia was administered. 1 gm of Ancef was given for infection prophylaxis. The patient was placed supine on the radiolucent table, with a bump under his right sacrum. A right thigh tourniquet was placed. The right leg was prepped from the toes to above the knee with alcohol and iodine. The leg was draped with an extremity drape. The leg was exanguinated, and the tourniquet inflated to 300 mm Hg. The fibula was approached first, using a 6 cm lateral incision centered over the fibula. As the patient is diabetic, great care was taken not to create unnecessary skin flaps. Care was taken to avoid the sural and superficial peroneal nerves. The fibula was exposed, and mini-Homan retractors were placed. The ends of the fracture were gently cleared of debris, and the fibula was reduced with a reduction clamp. A 16 mm 3.5 cortical lag screw was place from posterior to anterior, proximally to distally to stabilize the fracture, overdrilling the near fragment to create a lag effect. At this point, a 5 hole 1/3 tubular plate was used to neutralize the fracture, using two 14 mm cortical screws proximally and 2 fully threaded cancellous screws distally, 12 mm and 14mm. At this point, attention was turned to the medial malleolus.

A gently curved 4 cm incision was made over the medial malleolus. Care was taken to avoid the saphenous nerve and long saphenous vein. The fracture was visualized, and cleared of debris. A reduction clamp was used to effect an adequate reduction. A guide wire was used to hold the reduction, then over-drilled, and a 4-0 cannulated screw with a washer was inserted. The mini-C-arm was used to visualize the reduction, which was acceptable. The mortisse did not widen with external rotation, so a syndesmotic screw was not used. Both wounds were thoroughly irrigated, and closed with 2-0 proline far-near-near-far sutures. An adequately padded short leg cast was applied, and the patient went to PACU in stable condition.

Knee Arthroscopy—Meniscal Tear Dictation

The patient was brought to the operating room and placed under MAC anesthesia. The right knee was prepped with alcohol and betadine, and sterilely draped in the usual fashion. 2% lidocaine with epinephrine was injected subcutaneously into the portal sites. Standard three portal arthroscopy was performed. The patellofemoral joint was free from chondral damage. Going down the lateral gutter, no loose bodies were seen, and the popliteus tendon was intact. The lateral compartment had some grade 1 chondromalacia of the lateral tibial plateau. No meniscal tear was visualized. The ACL was intact in the notch. The medial joint showed a complex tear of the posterior horn of the medial meniscus, as well as a grade 4 osteochondral defect of the medial femoral condyle measuring 1.5 cm in diameter. The meniscal tear was in the white/white zone, and was irreparable. A partial menisectomy was performed with an upbiter and a shaver. The arthroscope was introduced carefully into the posterior compartment to visualize the attachment of the posterior horn of the medial meniscus and to make sure that the tear did not extend to the root. The PCL was visualized at this time and was intact. Attention was then turned to the OCD. A microfracture technique was performed on the OCD of the medial femoral condyle, using the 30 degree awl. The knee was then drained, and the portals were closed with 3-0 proline simple sutures. 20 cc of 0.25% marcaine with epinephrine was injected into the knee joint. A sterile dressing was applied, and the patient went to PACU in stable condition.

Operative Note

"A surgeon, an internist, and a pathologist went duck hunting. The internist went first. He thought as a bird flew by, 'Is this a duck? It has the characteristics of a duck, the distinguished, fluffy white feathers, the yellow bill. Ah, it just gave a distinctive quack, pathopneumonic for a duck.' By the time the internist decided to shoot, the duck had flown by. The surgeon was next. As a bird approached, he took a shotgun and blasted it. He turned to the pathologist and said, 'Could you pick that thing up and tell me what it is?'"

Every patient gets an operative note. Always include the operative findings, since the dictation often takes a few days. Always include all hardware placed in the procedure, including the brand. Get the post-operative plan from the attending and include it as well.

Pre-op diagnosis
Post-op diagnosis
Procedure (list all procedures)
Surgeon (the attending)
Assistants (residents, medical students)
Anesthesia: Local
MAC (monitored anesthesia care)
Epidural
Spinal
Regional Block (intra-scalene, femoral)
Combined
IVF (get from anesthesia)
EBL (get from anesthesia)
Drains (note if they are sutured in!)
Specimens
Complications (be sure to clear these with the attending)
Findings
Disposition (i.e. to PACU in stable condition)
Post-operative plan (weight-bearing, when drains are to be pulled, antibiotics, anti-coagulation)

Post-Op – Blood Products

Transfusions – Premedicate

Acetaminophen 650 mg PO.
Diphenhydramine 25 mg PO.
Split units when appropriate.
Consider diuretics between units, e.g. furosemide 20 mg IV.
Transfuse slowly if not for acute resuscitation.

Transfusions – Packed Red Cells

Single unit raises Hematocrit by 3%. Transfuse autologous blood if available.
Transfused typically over 3-4 hours per unit.

Indications
- Symptomatic anemia
- Large blood loss
- Relative <25% (some would say 21%)
- Consider lower limits in patients with chronic renal insufficiency
- Consider higher limits in patients with CAD, elderly, e.g. hct>30.

Transfusions – Platelets

Single unit raises count by 5000-10,000
Transfused typically 6 units at a time.

Indications:
- Relative <20K
- Less than 50K and bleeding or planned surgery
- Thrombocytopenia & NSAID & bleeding

Consider single donor in patients with history of multiple transfusions.
Consider CMV negative/irradiated in neutropenic patients.

FFP

Usually given as 1-2 units depending on PT and PTT.
Consider vitamin K 2-10 mg SQ if treating PT, but remember future anticoagulation will be difficult.

Cryoprecipitate

Only contains factor VIII, fibrinogen and von Wilbrand factor.
Consider use in patients with a deficiency of one or more of these specifically.

Post-Op – Blood Products (continued)

Transfusion reactions

Febrile, allergic, infectious (hepatitis C, CMV, HIV).

ARDs 2° donor WBC.

Volume overload.

Massive transfusions – dilutional thrombocytopenia, hyperkalemia, hypocalcemia, hypothermia.

Hemolytic transfusion reaction – fever, low back pain, nausea, chest discomfort, headache, hypotension, oliguria.

1. Stop transfusion.
2. Return blood with new specimen.
3. Get repeat X-match, Coombs.
4. Urine for free hemoglobin.
5. Support pressure – fluids, inotropes.
6. Watch for renal failure – furosemide or mannitol.

Post-Op DVT Prophylaxis

All patients are at risk of DVT. Virchow's triad: hypercoaguable states, prolonged immobility or stasis, and endothelial injury.

All ortho patients should get some DVT prophylaxis until they are ambulatory.

Options:

1. Compressive stockings with intermittent compression device (Ted's hose and SCD's)
2. Warfarin (must monitor INR, can take a few days to reach therapeutic level, some patients are extremely sensitive to warfarin and INR will jump quickly)
3. Low molecular weight heparins (no blood test to monitor, can have increased bleeding complications)
4. Heparin drip (not likely post-orthopaedic procedure as massive bleeding complications)

Bottom line: Most attendings are very specific on the type of anti-coagulation they prefer. CHECK!

Post-Op PUD Prophylaxis

Most likely necessary if patient is anticipated to be on steroids for a prolonged period of time.

Cushing's (brain trauma/pathology), Curling's (burn) and other stress related ulcers are prevented with the use of antacids, H-2 blockers or sucralfate. Sucralfate preserves gastric acidity and results in a decreased risk of colonization by more virulent flora. Choose from:

Sucralfate 1 gm PO bid.
Cimetidine 400 mg PO qHS.
Ranitidine 150 mg PO bid or 50 mg IV q 8° (renal adjustments needed).
Famotidine 20 mg PO bid or 20 mg IV bid.
Omeprazole 20 mg PO qd.
Protonix 40 mg PO/IV qd.

Post-Op Note

There should always be at least one post op note from after surgery and before rounds the next morning. Seniors and attendings do not like to be the first to be aware of a post-op problem!

Date and time
S/P (procedure)
S: How's the patient feel? Any complaints or abnormalities.
O: temperature, Vitals, drain output, urine output
Chest
Heart
Extremity: Neuro status, pulses, dressing status
A/P: pt is stable/unstable s/p procedure
Plan: Always put will d/w resident/attending for any unusual problems

Post-Op Care and Thoughts

Each day on every patient ask yourself:

1. Why does this patient have an IV?
2. Why is this patient on oxygen, and can I lower/discontinue it?
3. Should this patient be on antibiotics?
4. What are we doing for DVT prophylaxis?
5. Is this patient getting decubitus ulcers on heels or back?
6. Can I advance his/her diet?
7. Can any drugs be switched to po?
8. Is this patient getting out of bed?
9. How is this patient doing in P.T.?
10. When can I get the Foley/drain out?
11. Did I look at the wound today?
12. Is it time to remove the sutures/staples?
13. Why is this patient still in the hospital?
14. Do I need to talk to the resident? Social worker?

Post-Op Iatrogenesis Imperfecta

"Being paranoid, I'm rarely surprised."—Anonymous

Be vigilant. Here are a few iatrogenic items that bedevil the orthopaedic patient.

1. Fluid overload
2. Hypokalemia
3. Urosepsis from old Foley
4. Medication side effects when drugs are not adjusted for renal failure, hepatic failure, or advanced age.
5. Failure to recognize respiratory distress because it had been ignored by an earlier shift.
6. Failure to recognize sepsis because charted vital signs look better than the patient.
7. Wound infection in unmonitored surgical wounds.
8. Not considering pulmonary emboli or MI when the patient is having problems.
9. Heel/sacral decubitus ulcers.

Post-Op Drain Care

Orthopaedic surgeons are very particular about their drains. Get new instructions regarding drain care for each new patient. Remember, most orthopaedic surgeons do not suture in their drains unless there was an infection, so be careful when removing bandages if the plan is to keep the drain in place.

1. Straight drains. There is no suction applied to these. These are normally applied to more superficial areas. The Penrose is a typical example. Care sometimes involves slowly pulling the drain out sequentially over a couple days.
2. Suction drains. The Hemovac and Jackson-Pratt (JP) are typical examples. These can be put to self-suction (bulb) or to a vacuum source. These drains can clot off early in the post-op course. The tube can be gently milked or stripped to try to keep them open. **Do not push the tube back into the patient if it falls out.** Fenestrated drains should be cut between the holes when placed in the OR. This is to ensure that when the drain is removed and the end of the tube checked, the cut is between the fenestrations. If part of the drain breaks off in the patient, the break will be through the fenestration. If resistance is met while removing the drain, call the resident first to get instructions. They may have you attach traction to the drain, as the drain may have inadvertently been sutured in during closure.
3. Reinfusion drains. Typically after procedures that can have a large amount of blood loss post-op (Total hip replacement, total knee replacement). The blood retrieval system is self-contained and reinfused into the patient. This is set up in the OR. Each institution has specific protocols on when and how long after surgery the blood can be reinfused.
4. Chest tubes. Only chest tubes placed by orthopaedics (mainly spine surgery) should be removed by ortho. The dressing incorporates petroleum gauze to help maintain an airtight seal. A typical routine involves keeping the CT attached to 20 cm H20 until attending/resident indicates otherwise. Then it is placed to water seal. CXR's daily until the CT is d/c'd. Chest tubes are removed with a fair amount of gusto and after the patient has taken a full inspiration to help prevent the aspiration of air into the chest cavity. Check a CXR after pulling the tube.

Post-Op Advancing Diets

"Have you passed gas today?"

Most orthopaedic patients are started on clear liquids after major surgery and advanced to their regular diet as tolerated. If there has been major spine trauma/surgery or pelvic/acetabular surgery with an anterior approach, the patient may be initially NPO and slowly advanced as in general surgery abdominal cases. For these patients, ask, "Have you passed gas today? Have you had a bowel movement?" As the ileus resolves, with the colon coming back on line last, the diet is advanced. Most patients will be started on clear liquid sips. If sips are tolerated, the diet becomes clear liquids and the IV is heparin locked. Generally, most IV medications will be switched to oral within a day. After 24 hours of clears and passage of flatus, most patients are then advanced to a regular diet.

For any bump in the road, you generally fall back a step. If regular diet is not tolerated, try clears. If clears are not tolerated, it's back to the IV.

Post-Op Wound Care

"The ten most common causes of wound infection can be found attached to your hands."
—Richard Edlich, M.D., 1982.

Wound care is highly ritualized. It sounds obvious, but always wash your hands between patients (this is harder than you think on a busy service!). The operative dressing stays on until your senior tells you to take it off. For most cases, this is 48 hours after surgery. Once the surgical dressing is removed, normally a plain self-adhering bandage is sufficient. If the wound is soupy, the senior/attending may want betadine paint applied before each dressing change.

For wounds intentionally left open (infection), the technique of wet to dry dressings is used. To avoid overly enthusiastic application of saline, sometimes the term "moist" or "damp" to dry NS dressing is used. Gauze, moistened with saline, is packed within the wound and then removed q shift to debride the wound. Closure is then accomplished usually back in the O.R.

Some incisions, especially fasciotomies from compartment syndrome, are under too much tension to close immediately in the O.R. One strategy to avoid/lessen the need for skin grafting that may be employed is to use staples on the sides of the wound as posts and run a sterile rubber band through them. The ends are tied in knots that cannot go back through the staple. Daily, as the edema decreases, the ends are slowly brought together and new knots are tied. Do not touch the wound without sterile technique.

Post-Op Problems

Compartment Syndrome

This diagnosis requires a high index of suspicion and prompt management. Causes can be internal (bleeding, tissue edema into fascial compartments) or external (cast too tight). Be on the lookout for post-op patients requiring unusually high dosages of pain meds!

Remember the 5 P's of compartment syndrome:

Pain (out of proportion to injury)
Pallor (skin white or blue)
Paresthesias
Poikilothermia (cool extremity)
Pain with passive range of motion

You can often have palpable pulses in an extremity with compartment syndrome.

First step, remove all tight dressings/cast. If symptoms do not resolve, call for the compartment pressure monitor and call your senior for instructions. Compartment pressure measures above 30 mm Hg are diagnostic, but the conservative treatment with suspected compartment syndrome is fasciotomy in the O.R., not "wait and see."

Foot drop

Foot drop is caused by injury to the common peroneal nerve. Injury can be caused directly (laceration during lateral meniscal repair, tight dressing) or indirectly (manipulation during pelvic surgery, overlengthening a leg during total hip surgery). An absence of EHL/tibialis anterior function should be noted on the post op check. Then:

1. Loosen all dressings
2. Flex the knee to 45 degrees (decreases stress on common peroneal nerve)
3. Call your senior/attending

Post-Op Problems

Excessive post-op drainage

Orthopaedic procedures differ from general surgery procedures in that many cases are done under tourniquet control so some bleeding may only become evident post-op. Also, bone is very vascular, and procedures can have a lot of blood loss from bone oozing (total knee arthroplasty). 300-500 cc out by the first post-op check can be normal. In the immediate post-op period for more drainage,

1. Clamp the drain for an hour so that bleeding can tamponade itself;
2. Incrementally increase the drainage back to normal suction, usually over a period of 6 hours;
3. Check CBC, PT/PTT if patient anti-coagulated or malnourished;
4. Call your senior/attending

Deep Venous Thrombosis

The best method for treating DVT or PE is avoiding them altogether. Every orthopaedic patient should have consideration for DVT prophylaxis: Ted's hose and SCD's for all patients not fully ambulatory, warfarin or low molecular weight heparin. Stay away from heparin drips in post-op patients, if possible (excessive bleeding, wound dehiscence). The risk of a single DVT distal to the calf causing a PE is low (around 5%).

Risks (Virchow's triad)

- Stasis: immobility, obesity, CHF, pregnancy, general anesthesia
- Hypercoagulable state: malignancy, lupus anticoagulant factor
- Endothelial injury: trauma, venous insufficiency

Clinical evidence

- Unilateral leg swelling
- Leg pain/ calf tenderness
- Low-grade fever

Diagnosis

- Duplex U/S- good reliability, non-invasive
- Venogram-good for very proximal DVT's, invasive

Therapy

- Vascular consult usually
- Elevate lag
- Low Molecular Weight Heparin (LMWH)/Warfarin/heparin drip
  - Eg Lovenox 40 mg SCqD (up to 1 mg/kg/day)

ulmonary embolism

he clue to diagnosis is suspicion. No one sign or lab is completely reliable.

o not hesitate to get a pulmonary consult.

Vorkup tools include:
BG – often with respiratory alkalosis and/or hypoxia pO2<80.
KG, CXR, Doppler studies of LEs.
piral CT
Q scan, Pulmonary angiogram (gold standard).

herapy: oxygen.
Empiric heparin? Your resident should be on board for considering more aggressive measures.

leparin

5000 unit i.v. bolus is used to initiate therapy or to re-bolus if the PTT is still within normal range. Start continuous i.v. infusion at 1000 units/hr (20 or 25 units per hour depending on concentration.) If the patient is greater than 30 Kg consider beginning at 1200 units/hr.

The first PTT is collected 4-6 hours after the initial bolus and adjusted as ollows:

PTT	Bolus	Stop	Rate	Change	Repeat PTT
50	5000U	–	+3cc/hr	120/150U/hr*	6hrs
51–59	–	–	+2cc/hr	80/100U/hr	6hrs
60–85	–	–	none	–	next AM
86–95	–	–	–1cc/hr	40/50U/hr	next AM
96–120	–	30min	–2cc/hr	80/100U/hr	6hrs
120	–	60min	–3cc/hr	120/150U/hr	6hrs

When the PTT runs high, stay on top of wound and urine bleeding as well as checking stool guaiac, ng tube aspirate, and monitoring he hematocrit.

*e.g. a 120 unit per hour change for 20,000 units in 500cc or a 150 unit per hour change for 25,000 units in 500cc change.

Low Molecular weight Heparin may also be used (e.g. Lovenox 1 mg/kg SC q12°)

Post-Op Problems – Fever

Post-Op fever-5W's:

- Wind – atelectasis, pneumonia.
- Water – UTI.
- Wound – you must look at the wound.
- Walking – pulmonary embolus.
- Wonder drug – drug fevers.

When patients do not have an expected response to anti-infective regimens, think again about PE and undrained pus. Identify source:

- Blood cultures x 2.
- Urine for u/a, C&S.
- CXR.
- Other imaging.

Other cultural considerations:

- Blood cultures through central lines.
- Percutaneous drainage catheters.
- Pleural effusions.
- Ascites
- CSF
- Blisters
- Wounds/sinuses – usually very unhelpful.
- Any loculated collection the radiologist can reach.

Consider the high likelihood sources:

- Central lines
- Pulmonary
- Foley catheter
- Pulmonary emboli
- Heparin locks and IV
- Urinary tract
- Wounds
- Heart valves

Do you need:

- Antibiotics?

Culture everything first, BC x2, urine, sputum, all ports of all lines, any fluid collections.

- IV fluids?
- Further w/u?

Do you need an ID consult? Generally that decision is up to your resident and attending.

Post-Op Problems – Renal

Oliguria

Checklist:

1. Prerenal, renal, postrenal causes – several may be operative.
2. Flush the Foley.
3. Unless patient is clinically volume overloaded, begin with fluid boluses.
4. Consider immediately reversible processes:
   - Prerenal – fluids.
   - Infection.
   - Drugs.
   - Postrenal obstruction.
5. If the fluid challenge has not cleared up the diagnosis, check random serum and urinary Na*. Calculate a FENa. Diuretics cloud interpretation.
   - FENa* < 10 usually prerenal.
   - FENa* > 10 usually renal.
6. If the diagnosis is elusive, get a renal ultrasound early.
7. Consider a pulmonary artery catheter to check pressures and cardiac output.
8. Consider renal dopamine early.
9. Diuresis supports the Dx of prerenal.
10. Consider a renal consult.

Etiologies to consider:

- Prerenal:
  - Bleeding, bleeding, bleeding, bleeding!
  - Post–op
  - Sepsis
  - Pancreatitis
  - Small bowel obstruction
  - Burns
- Renal:
  - ATN – check CPK for rhabdomyolysis
- Postrenal:
  - Foley obstruction
  - Bilateral renal obstruction

Post-Op Problems – Cardiopulmonary

Chest Pain

If stable, i.e. normal vital signs, complete a brief w/u and let your resident know the results.
If unstable, initiate the workup and call your resident simultaneously.

In the category of common things being common, a cardiac source with angina and MI lead the differential. If the patient is lying in bed, anginal pain would often be considered unstable angina. Usual response to a patient with chest pain when considering cardiac origin:

- Nasal Oxygen at 2 liters.
- IV access.
- EKG stat.
- Give SL nitroglycerin after EKG.
- Start nitropaste 1-2 inches q 6 hours, hold MN to 6 AM.
- Consider cardiac enzymes to r/o MI.
- Consider lidocaine if frequent PVCs, Rs on T, polymorphic/multifocal PVCs.
- If EKG is suspicious and pain not relieved with 2-4 SL nitroglycerin:
    - Consider IV nitroglycerin.
    - ASA stat.
    - Call the ICU or CCU resident to arrange transfer.

Other diagnoses to consider: PE and aortic dissection are the first two thoughts!

Chest wall: rib fx, costochondral dislocation, costochondritis (Tietze syndrome), phlebitis (Mondor's syndrome).

Cardiac: if not MI, angina – stable or unstable, pericarditis, endocarditis.

Pulmonary: PE, pneumonia, pleurisy, pneumothorax (new lines?)

Esophageal: inflammation, spasm, rupture (Boerhaave's).

Aorta: dissection.

Subdiaphragmatic: abscess, cholecystitis, pancreatitis, dyspepsia.

Musculoskeletal – DJD, muscle strain, vertebral fracture, herpes zoster.

Post-Op Problems – Hypotension

Ask yourself, "Is the patient stable?" Look at the patient. Is the patient alert? It does not hurt to check the VS's yourself. Be wary of treating machine-generated numbers. Feel the groin (BP-60) and radial (BP-80) pulses yourself. Patients are often tolerant of low BP if kept flat.

IF THE PATIENT IS STABLE – then ask yourself, what did I do to this patient to make his or her blood pressure fall?

1. Is the patient bleeding from surgery? Is there any clinical evidence of bleeding? Is the patient stable enough to be imaged or will surgery be needed? Where is my resident?

2. New or increased medications: beta-blockers, calcium channel blockers, nitrates, morphine, sedatives.
   Think "rate, rhythm, preload, afterload, contractility."
   Reduce dose?
   Will a little preload help? 250cc NS IV over 1°.
   Do you need to do anything more than close observation?

3. s/p IV contrast – patients often are diuresing post dye load.
   Think "rate, rhythm, preload, afterload, contractility."
   Try preload, 250 – 500cc NS IV over 1°.

4. Dopamine running into bed instead of patient.
   Replace IV.

IF THE PATIENT IS UNSTABLE, again, ask yourself "Why?" Get help. Consider a general surgery, internal medicine, or ICU consult.

Is it "rate, rhythm, preload, afterload, or contractility"? Be sure your patient is not in failure. If the lungs are clear, remember volume is usually very effective. Sick patients are much trickier to handle before they code (it's cookbook after the code starts). Get some help.

First think about the basics. Be thorough and systematic; in unstable patients, it is important not to be distracted by the first abnormal physical finding you run across. If possible, find the chart and the drug list. Look for drugs that cause hypotension that you can stop, e.g. nitropaste, blood pressure medications, etc. Correct hypoglycemia (D50) and reverse narcosis (naloxone 2 mg) early.

Post-Op Problems – Hypotension (continued)

1. Have your resident paged.
2. ABC – Airway, Breathing, Circulation. Get new VS's, do you need to call a code?
3. Call for EKG, portable CXR, and respiratory therapy, 100% O_2, ABG.
4. Establish IV, send labs: glucose, Lytes, Ca**, Mg**, CBC, and open up the saline.
5. Concentrate on the Elements of Circulation:

Rate – Effective 60 – 130. If symptomatic bradycardia, consider pacing transvenous or transcutaneous, atropine, or isoproterenol. If pacemaker already present turn up to 100.

Rhythm - Sinus is best. Is a rhythm change part of the problem? Fast rates and unstable need electricity, cardioversion. If ventricular rate is between 60 and 130, cardioversion is unlikely to be helpful. Do not give calcium channel blockers to hypotensive patients or patients with wide complex tachycardia. Consider adenosine for PSVT and digoxin for aftib/aflutter.

Preload – Fill the pump before whipping it. Volume!
IV – NS bolus or wide open
Use neck veins, lung exam, S3, CXR, swan as your guide
Consider SPA in your volume-overloaded intravascularly-dry patient.

Afterload – May be impossible to judge without a PA catheter. Dopamine is the fist line agent because it enhances both afterload and contractility. Afterload is increased with norepinephrine, epinephrine, and Neo-Synephrine as well. Increasing the afterload increases the cardiac work. {Interventions that decrease afterload are: balloon pump, renal dose dopamine, dobutamine, hydralazine, nitroprusside, nitroblycerin, and Inocor (amrinone).}

Contractility – Correct acidosis, inotropics – dobutamine, Inocor, calcium. Often the combination of increasing contractility and dropping afterload will improve perfusion to kidneys and other vital organs.

Use ACLS protocols for Asystole, Bradycardia, PEA, Vfib, and Vtach.
If no pulse start CPR.

Post-Op Problems – Hypertension

Check orders. Was a medication that the patient usually takes stopped?

End-organ symptoms represent an emergency – Neuro, Cardiac, or Renal.

Treat underlying pain, agitation, DTs, hypoxia first. Be careful in the setting of recent neurologic events, the brain may need that elevated pressure. Also be careful in the setting of polypharmacy.

Isolated HTN – Maximize current blood pressure medications.

Clonidine 0.2mg PO repeat with 0.1mg q1° as necessary (works in 30 min – 2 hours, watch for rebound and orthostatics).

Nitropaste 1" topically.

Nitroglycerin IV –	venodilator	30 ug/min
	arteriodilator	>150 ug/min

Nitroprusside 0.5 – 30 ug/min is a very effective arterial vasodilator.

Labetalol can be used IV and later switched to PO.

NB: Chronically hypertensive patients are often volume depleted and may crash from hypertensive to hypotensive with therapy. Keep an eye on K^{+} and Mg^{++}.

Post-Op Problems – Short-of-breath

Dyspnea is never a complaint to manage over the phone. It may be anxiety, but you need to decide that in person. Ask yourself, is this an acute event or an exacerbation of a pre-existing condition, e.g. COPD, pneumonia, asthma. What is the patient's baseline cardiac and pulmonary function? Are they on any respiratory or cardiac medications?

Think about the biggies:

Hypervolemia and CHF.
MI and CHF.
Acute renal failure and CHF.
Bronchial plugging.
Pulmonary embolus.
Bronchospasm.
Pneumonia.
Aspiration.
Pneumothorax.
COPD exacerbation.
Anaphylaxis.

Quick history – What was the patient doing when it started?

Acute or subacute?
Pleuritic component? Chest pain?
Cardiac history? Pulmonary history? Smoker?
Current medications?
Are they currently on oxygen? At home?

Physical exam-

General: comfort, diaphoresis, able to talk.
Neck: +/- JVD.
Chest: stridor, rales, rhonchi, wheezing, equal breath sounds, diminished or absent breath sounds.
Cor: rhythm, murmur, gallops, pulsus paradoxus.
Ext: edema (unilateral or bilateral), cyanosis.

Post-Op Problems – Short-of-breath (continued)

Consider:

- Pulse ox, ABG, EKG, portable CXR.
- 100% O2 face mask (with the COPD as the exception).
- Calling your resident.
- Calling anesthesia.
- Respiratory therapy.
- Wall suction, intubation tray.
- Nasotracheal suction.
- Thoracotomy tray.
- For failure, see page 47, nitrates, morphine, oxygen.
- For asthma, consider:
  - Proventril nebulizer treatments
  - Hydrocortisone 100 mg IV.
  - Aminophylline drip 6 mg/kg IV over 30 min then 0.4-0.9 mg/kg/hour.

For pulmonary embolus, see page 33. Have a high index of suspicion.

If you have trouble getting the help you need, call a code. That will produce a room full of consultants and facilitate transfer to the appropriate intensive care unit.

Post-Op – Disasters

"The method by heart compression has proved to be of great value in many cases of chloroform syncope. Success is denoted by artificially produced carotid pulse and contraction of pupils, which should control the force and rapidity of impulses."—Joseph Bryant, M.D., 1905.

Anticipate disaster, it lurks in the coronaries and deep leg veins of every patient.
Hypoxia follows aspiration which follows sedation every day. Even the healthiest of patients can get staphylococcal sepsis from their heparin lock.

Checklist –

1. Call your resident.
2. Call the attending.
3. Call the family.

Ideally, your resident should call the attending early with a disaster report with workup in progress. It gets everybody into the same boat and saves on the day after clairvoyance.

Ortho Topics – ATLS in Brief

Prior to Arrival: The team should include a captain, one or two other physicians capable of carrying out any necessary procedures, two RNs, an anesthesiologist, RT, and X-ray techs. Consider mechanism of injury, VSs, mental status in field, and transport time. Have airway equipment, chest tubes and line kits ready at the bedside.

I. Primary Survey: Team captain calls out findings.

Airway with Cervical Spine Stabilization: chin-lift and jaw thrust without head tilt. Maintain in-line cervical stabilization with collar and assistant during all maneuvers. Suction blood or secretions and remove debris. Intubate PRN.

Breathing: Assess rate and depth. Inspect for open wounds, flail chest, distended neck veins, and tracheal deviation. Auscultate for equal breath sounds. Palpate for crepitus, rib fractures, subcutaneous air. Reassess need to intubate and insert chest tubes prior to CXR if any doubt.

Circulation: Control external hemorrhage with direct pressure. Check pulses. Pulse rate is good indication of volume status Note skin perfusion.

- Carotid Palpable: SBP > 60
- Femoral Palpable: SBP > 70
- Radial Palpable: SBP > 80

Consider occult hemorrhage:

- Examine abdomen for tenderness and bowel sounds.
- Rock pelvis and press down and in on iliac spines.

Deficit: Brief mental status=AVPU (Alert, responds to Voice, responds to Pain, Unresponsive.)

- Pupils for reaction and symmetry.
- Moves all 4 extremities.

Exposure: Completely undress patient, log-roll penetrating trauma patients early.

II. Resuscitation: Concomitant with primary survey.

O_2: 100% administered initially.
IV Access: 2 or more short 14-16 G IVs then one or more EtOH, Tox Screen.

IVF: Ringer's or NS for first 2 liters initially. 20 ml/kg initial bolus in children. Once initial bolus exhausted, begin with blood as available: Type O-(stat), Type specific (ten minutes), crossmatched (20-30 minutes).
Monitors: Cardiac, pulse-ox, BP.

"Finger or tube in every orifice":
Rectal: Inspect for tone, saddle anesthesia, boggy or high riding prostate, guaiac.
Foley: Check for prostate injury, scrotal hematoma, or blood at meatus first.
III. Secondary Survey: includes radiography and constant re-evaluation of the patient.

A. Neurologic: Glasgow Coma Scale GCS (3-15)

Eye opening (E)	
Spontaneous	4
To Loud Voice	3
To Pain	2
Nil	1
Motor Response (M)	
Obeys Verbal Command	6
Localizes Pain	5
Flexion Withdrawal	4
Decorticate rigidity	3
Decerebrate rigidity	2
Nil	1
Verbal Response (V)	
Oriented/converses	5
Disoriented/converses	4
Inappropriate words	3
Incomprehensible	2
Nil	1

Inspect pupils for reaction and symmetry, cranial nerves, tympanic membranes and peripheral nerves.

B. Head to Toe exam:

Scalp: hematomas, lacerations, skull fractures.
Face: orbital rims, zygomas, nasal bones, septal hematoma, maxilla fractures (leFort). Mandible fractures.
Neck: tenderness, crepitus, neck veins, wounds, hematomas.
Chest: reassess.
Heart: diminished sounds, murmurs.
Abdomen: contusions, hematomas, scars, tenderness, bowel sounds
Genitalia: penis, scrotum, bimanual in women, hematuria.
Back: spinous tenderness, lacerations, abrasions.
Extremities: deformity, tenderness, crepitus.

C. Radiology:

C-spine: must visualize C1 to top of T1. Cross table lateral first, then swimmer's if needed, follow-up with AP and odontoid view after stabilization complete.
Chest: r/o PTX, hemothorax.
AP Pelvis.
T-spine and LS-spine generally after stabilization unless suspected injury exists.
Head CT.
Abdominopelvic CT.

Ortho Topics – Suture Material

You will likely have little autonomy in terms of choosing suture material (it will be up to the attending). Nevertheless, one day someone will ask you what you want, and it is worthwhile to know the basic choices.

In general:

1. In most situations, choose an absorbable suture. A non-absorbable monofilament suture is used if scarring poses a problem.
2. Definitely absorbable if infection is present.
3. Nonabsorbable suture with high tensile strength is used for fascial cover.
4. Nonabsorbable suture with high tensile strength is also used when strength is necessary over long periods of time, i.e., vascular anastomosis.
5. The attending or resident's choice is always the right one.

Type of suture	Tensile strength	Absorption Rate	Reaction
Absorbable suture material			
plain		0% 7-10 days	70 days
moderate			
chromic	0% 21-28	90 days	moderate
Vicryl (polygalactin)	65% 21-28	70 days	mild
PDS (monofilament)	85%-wks	210 days	slight
Silk (braided)	0%-1 year	2 years	moderate
Nonabsorbable suture material			
cotton	50% decrease at 6 mos		minimal
steel	indefinite		minimal
Ethilon (nylon)	decrease 15% year low		
Nurolon	decrease 15%		very low
Mersilene (braided polyester)	indefinite		minimal
Ethibond (braided polyester)	indefinite		minimal
Prolene (monofilament)	indefinite		minimal

Ortho Topics – Casting/Splinting

Casting is an art, and proficiency comes with practice. It's beyond the scope of this book to teach casting, but here are some hints.

1. If the attending wants a long leg/long arm cast, take it as high as you can. "If a long leg cast doesn't catch some pubic hair, it's not high enough."
2. If the cast is being used to hold a reduction, plaster is better than fiberglass. Plaster can be molded and shaped as it hardens.
3. Fiberglass is lighter than plaster and more water-resistant. If you wish to use fiberglass but need to hold a reduction, consider using a thin wrap of plaster, let it harden in the position that you want, and then reinforce with fiberglass. Never handle fiberglass without gloves.
4. When rubbing the fiberglass to shape and smooth it, soap/hand lotion on your gloves is helpful so your gloves won't stick to the cast. Alternatively, you can wrap a soaking wet ACE wrap around the cast, then smooth the cast. Unwrap the ACE after it is set.
5. The cotton webril serves two purposes. It protects the skin from the heat of the cast hardening, and it protects the skin from the cast saw. The more webril applied, the harder it is to hold a reduction.
6. When taking off a cast with a cast saw, do not saw through the cast longitudinally, or you can "stripe" the patient's skin. The cast saw vibrates to cut, so if you push straight down perpendicular to the cast, come back up, and repeat a half inch down, you can safely remove the cast.
7. Elbow splints should initially extend past the wrist like an ulnar gutter splint. This gives better immobilization of the elbow and less pain.

Ortho Topics – Septic Joint

When asked to see a patient for evaluation of a possible septic joint, there are important points in the history to consider.

1. Constitutional symptoms
2. Prior history of pain in this joint or other painful joints
3. Prior history of trauma to this joint
4. History of rheumatoid arthritis or other related diseases (Lupus, Reiter's)
5. Immune competency (malignancy, HIV, chronic steroids, prior transplant, diabetes)
6. IV drug abuse

With infants, the index of suspicion must be high since the only symptoms may be failure to thrive, irritability, or infection at another site.

Whenever possible, aspirate the joint before starting antibiotics.
For aspiration, widely prep the skin with betadine, numb the skin with a small-bore needle with 1% plain lidocaine, then aspirate with a large bore needle. Avoid puncturing skin through areas of cellulitis.

Send fluid for Gram stain, culture, cell count, and crystal analysis. Synovial cell counts of greater than 50,000 is a positive indicator of septic arthritis, but a lower count does not necessarily preclude it.
Send peripheral blood for WBC, erythrocyte sedimentation rate (ESR) and C-reactive protein (CRP).

Aspiration of Common Joints

Ankle-Insert needle 2.5 cm proximal and 1.3 cm anterior to tip of lateral malleolus.

Knee-With knee bent at 90 degrees, insert needle 1 cm distal and 1 cm lateral to distal pole of patella, aiming for the intercondylar notch Alternatively, with the knee extended, insert needle laterally underneath the superior Patella.

Hip-Requires fluoroscopy unless in skilled hands.

Shoulder-Insert needle anteriorly at midpoint between coracoid and anterlateral edge of acromion, aiming posteriorly.

Elbow-Aim needle at the soft spot between lateral epicondyle, radial head, and olecrenon. The needle will go through anconeous.

Common Organisms:

Newborns-Staph aureus and Group B strep

3 months to 15 years-Staph aureus, Strep pneumoniae, and Hempohilus influenzae (decreased with vaccine)

Adults-Neisseria gonorrhoeae, S. aureus, strep

Ortho Topics – Child Abuse

When called to do a consult on a child with a fracture, always have a diagnosis of abuse in the back of your mind, because if you don't think about it, you will miss it. Do not assume that someone else must have thought about it.

Incidence—15 per 1000 children
Prevalence—42 per 1000 children
Abuse 2nd to SIDS as cause of death of infants 1–6 months old
Abuse 2nd to accidents as cause of death in children <1 year

Clinical signs—Often children overly passive or aggressive, hyperactive, or developmentally delayed
—parents/caregivers may
1. Give vague histories
2. Delay seeking care
3. Be hostile or casual to questioning
4. Give contradictory histories

Radiologic signs—Best indicator is multiple fx's in various stages of healing.
Most often fx's are diaphyseal.
Metaphyseal fx's ("Corner Fx's") are more specific for child abuse.

Be tactful with caregivers, but report it immediately, either by calling social worker/Child Protective Services or bring to attention of E.D./pediatric attending.

Documentation of your exam is critical in the consult—include all findings and patient/caregiver comments.

Fracture Conference – Pearls for Survival

Nothing can be more intimidating to a new orthopaedic resident than fracture conference. It can sometimes feel like "Wild Kingdom" where you're the llama that has strayed from the pack, facing a group of hungry lions. The best way to prepare is to find out ahead of time the cases that are to be presented and read about them. Start with the basics (anatomy, physical exam, fracture classification). If you read advanced treatments in the latest journal article but don't know the basics, it will look like you didn't prepare at all, because the questions usually start easy and, as you answer them, get more advanced.

When called to do a case, stand straight and not directly in front of the X-rays. Do not stuff your hands in your pockets. If allowed to get a history, ask for it. Especially important is mechanism, open injury, neurovascular status, and associated injuries. This can also clue you in to what to look for on X-ray and buy time. When reading X-rays aloud, always start with what X-rays are shown and of what and in whom. For example, "This is an A/P, Lateral, and Mortisse view of a right ankle in a skeletally mature individual." If you can't figure out what exact views are shown, an alternative is, "This is a right ankle series in a skeletally mature individual."

Try to answer questions directly. Do not offer unsolicited information unless you're thoroughly prepared to delve into this side avenue in detail. If you don't know an answer, say so. Non-operative treatment is always an option, but may not be a good option. NEVER argue with the presenter or the audience. Sometimes, what you've read may be different than what the attendings or the seniors believe. You can graciously point this out that you specifically read something different, but do it humbly. These conferences can be the attendings' only contact with you for some time, and many reputations (good and bad) are made here.

Included in the following pages are some ammunition for questions commonly asked of beginning orthopaedic residents.

The following pages are not an exhaustive discussion on orthropedics, they are more on assembly of common questions used to assess the intellectual development of orthopaedic residents.

Fracture Conference – Internal Fixation

Cortical screw-fully threaded-designed to "bite" opposite cortex-since fully threaded, does not compress.

Cancellous screw-larger threads for purchase in metaphyseal bone-if partially threaded, will create a "lag effect" (compress) by pulling far fragment toward the near fragment.

Lag screw-Either a partially threaded cancellous screw where the threaded portion pulls the far fragment in OR a cortical screw where the near fragment was drilled to a larger diameter than the threaded screw.

Compression plate-plate applied with screws placed asymmetrically in the screw holes away from the fracture, thereby tensioning the plate and compressing the fracture.

Neutralization plate-counteracts torsion, bending and shear-does not compress fracture.

Buttress plate-counteracts compression and shear for epiphyseal/metaphyseal fx's-plate often not attached to fragment it is supporting.

Bridge plate-spans a comminuted fx, often applied with little periosteal dissection to maximize healing.

Blade plate-plate with an angled (usually 95 degrees) spike designed to hold in metaphyseal bone-advantage over 95 degree dynamic condylar screw plate is that there is less bone loss when putting in the slim blade and the blade better controls rotation.

Dynamic condyular screw plate-screw can hold in metaphyseal bone-advantage over blade plate is the ease of insertion (more user friendly).

Locking plate-new-the screws actually lock into the plate, creating a rigid construct without getting a cortical bite on the opposite side with the screw. With nonlocking plates, the screw slides, compressing the plate against the bone.

Intramedullary Nails

1st Generation (unlocked)-nail acts as a scaffold.

2nd Generation (locked nails)-most rigid nails are locked at least on one side of a weightbearing limb-Nail is "dynamic" if locked on one side of fracture and the other bone end is free to slide with weightbearing, compressing the fracture. Nail is "static" if both sides are locked and fracture cannot compress.

3rd Generation (cephalomedullary nail)-Proximal fragment in femur is locked with cancellous screws into the femoral head.

External Fixation

Good for open fx's, fx's with severe soft tissue compromise, and fx's with bone loss or severe comminution.

Simple frame-half pins into bone on both sides of fracture, attached to rods.

Hybrid frame-half pins on one side, tensioned wires applied to a circular frame on the other side (usually near a joint surface).

Ilizarov frame-circular frame and tensioned wires on both sides, usually used when angular, rotational, or length deformities need to be gradually corrected, 1 mm a day (0.25 mm four times a day).

Hip

Blood supply to femoral head is mainly from the lateral epiphyseal artery, the terminal branch of the medial femoral circumflex artery.

Femoral Neck Fractures-

Garden classification

Type I-incomplete fracture or VALGUS impacted fx.

Type II-non-displaced, fracture completely through neck.

Type III-displaced, trabecular pattern from head to shaft do not line up.

Type IV-displaced, trabecular pattern from head to shaft line up (2 completely separate fragments).

Alternatively, Type I-II are stable fractures, Type III/IV are unstable. Any fracture in varus is unstable.

Non-displaced fractures are amenable to percutaneous pinning.

Displaced fractures need ORIF or hemiarthroplasty.

More likely to use hemiarthroplasty if the patient is older (physiologic age >70), cannot be reliable to be NWB or TTWB, or the longer the time was from injury to surgery (osteonecrosis of femoral head).

Fracture Conference – Hip

Approach	Interval	Danger
Posterior (Moore)	Muscle split of gluteus maximus	Sciatic nerve, if not protected by short external rotators Inferior gluteal artery
Anterolateral (Watson-Jones)	Tensor fascia and gluteus medius	Superior gluteal nerve Lateral femoral circumflex artery
Anterior (Smith-Peterson)	Tensor fascia femoris and satorius	Lateral femoral cutaneous nerve (meralgia paresthetica)
Lateral (Hardinge)	Gluteus medius/vastus lateralis split	Femoral nerve Superior gluteal nerve
Medial (Ludloff)-(Pediatric)	Adductor longus and gracilis Adductor brevis and magnus	Obturator nerve Medial femoral circumflex artery

Intertrochanteric Hip Fractures are below femoral neck and involve the greater/lesser trochanter.

Classification –

Two part-through greater and lesser trochanter.

Three part – same fracture pattern as two part with a separate greater/lesser trochanter piece.

Four part – with separate greater and lesser trochanter pieces.

Reverse obliquity-high energy injury, more likely in younger patients from MVA.

The higher the energy injury, the more pieces. Usually with three/four part fractures, there will be posteromedial comminution.

Treatment – ORIF with a sliding hip screw (ex. DHS) or intramedullary device.

For reverse obliquity, use either an intramedullary device or a 95 degree fixed angle device (blade plate or screw).

Subtrochanteric Hip Fracture – fractures that start and end from lesser trochanter to 5 cm distal to lesser trochanter.

Russell-Taylor classification –

Type 1A – no extension into piriformis fossa and or lesser trochanter (can use intramedullary nail with standard locking).
Type 1B – no extension into piriformis fossa, fracture includes lesser trochanter (needs a cephalomedullary nail that has a screw into the femoral head).
Type 2 – extension into the greater trochanter and piriformis fossa (best choice-95 degree device with possible bone grafting).

Femoral Head Fractures

These fractures are usually sustained after fracture/dislocation of the hip.

Pipkin Classification

Type I–posterior dislocation with fracture caudad to fovea centralis.
Type II–posterior dislocation with fracture cephalad to fovea centralis.
Type III–Type I or II with associated femoral neck fracture.
Type IV–Type I–II with associated acetabular fracture.

Femoral head fractures can cause a hip fracture to be irreducible (fragment in joint).

Acetabular Fractures

Classified by Letournel and Judet

Simple Types	Complex Types
Posterior Wall	T-Type
Posterior Column	Posterior Column/Posterior Wall
Anterior Wall	Transverse/Posterior Wall
Anterior Column	Anterior Column/Posterior Hemi-transverse
Transverse	Both Columns

Fracture Conference – Hip, Pelvis

Approaches

Kocher-Langebeck-good for posterior wall, posterior column, posterior wall/posterior column, and some transverse fractures.

Ilioinguinal-good for anterior wall, anterior column and some transverse fractures.

Some fractures may require a combined anterior/posterior approach or an extensile exposure such as an iliofemoral or triradiate approach.

Pelvic Fractures

The pelvis is comprised of the ilium, ischium and pubis. It is joined to the sacrum posteriorly through the sacroiliac (SI) joints posteriorly and the pubic symphysis anteriorly. The acetabulum is formed by the fusion of these three bones at the triradiate cartilage.

Structures that run through the greater sciatic foramen (including the piriformis):

Above Piriformis:	Superior Gluteal Artery and Nerve
Below Piriformis:	Inferior Gluteal Artery and Nerve
	Internal Pudendal Artery
	Sciatic Nerve
	Pudendal Nerve
	Posterior Femoral Cutaneous Nerve
	Nerve to Quadratus Femoris
	Nerve to Obturator Externus

On X-ray, the inlet view (beam is 40 degrees cephalad looking caudad) demonstatres anterior-posterior displacement of SI joints and pelvis. The outlet view (beam is 25 degrees caudad looking cephalad) demonstrates vertical displacement.

Urogenital, lumbosacral plexus, and intra-abdominal injuries as well as other long bone fractures are commonly encountered as these fractures are frequently the result of high energy trauma.

Young Classification divides pelvic fractures into 4 types:

- Lateral Compression (LC)-examples are iliac wing fractures and pubic rami fractures.
- Anteroposterior Compression (APC)-longitudinal pubic symphysis diastasis such as an open book fracture.

- Vertical Shear (VS)-pubic symphysis displacement in a cephalad-caudad direction.
- Combined Mechanism (CM)-combination of injury patterns with LC/VS most common of these.

Treatment-Stable fractures can be observed with early weight bearing. Unstable fractures (including those with obvious fracture gapping, disruption of posterior SI joints, or pubic symphysis diastasis greater than 3 cm) may require fixation such as percutaneous SI screws, anterior plating, or external fixation.

Femur

X-rays should always include the hip and knee (10% incidence of femoral neck fractures with femoral shaft fractures).

Can classify by Winquist/Hansen classification (used to determine if distal locking necessary).

- Type O-no butterfly fragment
- Type I – inconsequential butterfly fragment
- Type II – >50% intact cortical contact
- Type III – <50% intact cortical contact
- Type IV – no intact cortical contact (highly comminuted)
- Type V – segmental

At the board, the best way is just to describe what you see: "Mid-third femoral shaft fracture with a large butterfly fragment."

Treatment-Normally intramedullary nailing. If asked, lock the nail both proximally and distally (safest bet).

Early nailing (within 24 hrs) decreases pulmonary complications.

Knee

<u>Femoral Condyle Fractures</u>-

AO classification

- A-extra-articular
- B-single condyle involved
- C-intra-articular with both condyles involved

Treatment is usually a 95 degree blade plate or screw, or a retrograde IM nail.

Fracture Conference – Knee, Ankle

Patella Fractures-Most fractures are longitudinal. Vertical fractures are best seen on sunrise view. Non-displaced fractures can be treated in extension casting. Displaced fractures (2 mm of articular step-off, 3 mm of cortical separation) are candidates for ORIF.

Tibial Plateau Fractures-

Shatzker Classification-

Type I – Lateral split
Type II – Lateral split/depression
Type III – Lateral pure depression
Type IV – Medial tibial plateau fx
Type V – Bicondylar fx with intact metaphysis
Type VI – Bicondylar fx with metaphyseal/diaphyseal dissociation

Treatments include non-operative for non-displaced fx's, perc pinning, ex-fix, hybrid ex-fix, ORIF with plating (risk of double plating for Type V/VI fx is AVN from periosteal stripping).

Pes Anserine muscles-"Say Grace before Tea For Our Souls" – Sartorius (Femoral Nerve), Gracilis (Obturator Nerve), Semitendinosis (Sciatic Nerve)

Tibial Shaft Fractures-

Normally classified by location (proximal/middle/distal third) and appearance (spiral, oblique, transverse).

Criteria for acceptable treatment with long leg cast after closed reduction: <5 degrees varus/valgus malalignment, <10 degrees anteroposterior malalignment, <10 degrees rotational malalignment, and <15 mm shortening.

Even if treatment is casting, consider overnight admission to watch for compartment syndrome!

For many tibia fractures, treatment of choice is IM rod.

For distal tibial shaft fractures, may need ORIF (no room distally to the lock the rod).

Ankle

X-ray views are A/P, lateral, and mortisse views (mortisse is best to look for widening-the clear space should be symmetric from superior surface of the tibiotalar joint to the space between the medial malleolus to the talus).

Fracture Conference – Ankle

Classifications –

Weber classification is easiest and based on the fibula.

Type A – fracture is distal the tibiotalar joint.
Type B – fracture is at the level of the tibiotalar joint.
Type C – fracture is above the tibiotalar joint.

Lauge – Hansen classification more complicated-based on ligaments of ankle and cadaver studies.

Supination-Adduction (SAD) – low Weber A fx of fibula with vertical medial malleolus fx.

Supination-External Rotation (SER) – spiral Weber B fx of fibula starting anteroinferior going posterosuperior with oblique medial malleolus fx.

Pronation-External Rotation (PER) – short spiral high Weber C fx starting posteroinferior going anterosuperior (opposite of SER) with medial malleolus fx.

Pronation-Abduction (PAB) – transverse Weber C fx and transverse avulsion fx of medial malleolus.

Treatment-ORIF if fibula is significantly displaced and/or the patient has MEDIAL tenderness (deltoid ligament injury) – Fix both the fibula and medial malleolus if fractured–Weber C fractures may require a syndesmotic screw.

Maissoneauve fx – medical malleolus fx with *proximal* fx.

Ankle sprain – lateral side (Anterior talofibular ligament), medial side (deltoid ligament), "high" ankle sprain (Syndesmotic injury, can take twice as long to heal as other sprains).

Ottawa Ankle rules – to determine if X-rays necessary–no substitute for clinical judgment.

1. Age >35
2. Inability to take four steps in E.D.
3. Tender to palpation over either malleolus

<u>Talar Neck Fractures</u> (Aviator's Astragalus)

Hawkin's classification useful for determining risk of osteonecrosis.

Fracture Conference – Ankle, Wrist

Type I – non-displaced fx-AVN risk 0–13%
Type II – fx with subtalar dislocation-AVN risk 20–50%
Type III – Type II fx with tibiotalar dislocation-AVN risk 80–100%
Type IV–rare-fx with talonavicular dislocation
Try to use titanium screws so that post-op MRI possible to look for AVN.

Hawkin's sign-talar subchondral radiolucency on X-ray 6–8 weeks post injury – This is a good sign demonstrating adequate blood supply and low risk of osteonecrosis.

"Tom, Dick, and A Very Nervous Harry" – mnemonic for structures behind medial malleolus going anterior to posterior (Tibialis Posterior, Flexor Digitorum Longus, Posterior Tibial Artery, Vein, Nerve, Flexor Hallucis Longus).

Os Trigonum-accessory bone at posterior and plantar talus-can cause compression of Posterior Tibial Nerve (Tarsal Tunnel Syndrome).

Wrist

Wrist fractures are the most common orthopaedic injuries.

Frykman Classification:

I – no intra-articular extension
II – I with ulnar styloid fx
III – radiocarpal extension
IV – III with ulnar styloid fx
V – radioulnar joint extension
VI – V with ulnar styloid fx
VII – both radiocarpal and radioulnar joint extension
VIII – VII with ulnar styloid fx

Eponyms:

Colles' fx: with dorsal displacement (apex of the fracture is volar; most common).
Smith's fx: with volar displacement (apex is dorsal).
Barton's fx: dislocation of the carpus on the radius.
Chauffeur's fx: Radial styloid fx.
Die-punch fx: lunate fossa impaction fx.

Other Hand/Upper extremity Epnoyms: Monteggia fx (ulnar shaft fracture with radial head dislocation), Galeazzi fx (distal third radial shaft fx with DRUJ dislocation), Gamekeeper's or Skier's thumb (insufficiency of ulnar collateral ligament of thumb), and Kienbock's disease (Avascular necrosis of the lunate).

It is imperative to do a thorough neurovascular exam upon initial evaluation and after casting. Swelling or extreme flexion with casting can cause median nerve compression.

X-rays: P/A film to assess radial length (normal 11 mm) and radial inclination (normal 22 degrees). Lateral film to assess volar tilt (normal 11 degrees) ("11/22/11" rule).

Criteria for acceptable reduction: Change in palmar tilt <10 degrees, radial shortening <2 mm, <1–2 mm of articular step off.

First treatment can usually be a cast – Final definitive fixation may be casting, perc pinning and casting, ex-fix, or plating.

Bones of the Carpus (Some Lovers Try Positions That They Can't Handle) – Scaphoid, Lunate, Triquetrum, Pisiform, Trapezium, Trapezoid, Capitate, Hamate.

Scaphoid – major blood supply from radial artery, entering dorsal ridge-blood supply distal to proximal-any step-off makes scaphoid fx unstable (ORIF with possible bone grafting).

Dorsal compartments of the wrist from thumb to little finger (I Abductor pollicis longus, Extensor pollicis brevis; II Ext. Carpi Radialis longus, ECRB; III Ext. pollicis longus; IV Ext. indicis, extensor digitorum communis; V Ext. digiti minimi; VI Ext. carpi ulnaris).

Elbow

Most distal humerus fractures in adults require ORIF. An olecrenon osteotomy affords the best visualization.

Capitellum Fx's –

Type I – complete fx of capitellum with large bone fragment (Hahn-Steinthal I).
Type II – thin osteochondral fragment (Kocher-Lorenz).

Type III – comminuted.
Type IV – fracture line extends into trochlea past lateral trochlear ridge (Hahn-Steinthal II).

Radial Head Fx's –

Mason classification:

- Type I – non-displaced.
- Type II – displaced fragment.
- Type III – comminuted.
- Type IV – fx with dislocation.

ORIF for Types II–IV

Beware the Essex – Lopresti lesion (injury to interosseous ligament can be seen with radial head fx's).

Coronoid Fx's –

- Type I – tip of coronoid – usually stable-only indication for surgery if loose body develops.
- Type II – <50% coronoid involvement – can contribute to elbow instability.
- Type III – >50% coronoid involvement – often associated with elbow instability.

Tennis Elbow (Lateral elbow tendinosis) – tendinosis of ECRB.

Golfer's Elbow (Medial elbow tendinosis) – tendinosis of PT/FCR.

Country Club Elbow – both tennis elbow and golfer's elbow.

Pediatrics

Salter Classification for fractures of the Physis in the skeletally immature.

- Type I – fx through the physis.
- Type II – fx line through physis with metaphyseal fragment.
- Type III – fx line through physis with epiphyseal fragment.
- Type IV – fx with both metaphyseal and epiphyseal fragments.
- Type V – crush injury to physis.

Pediatric Elbow

Pediatric elbow mnemonic for remembering the appearance of ossification centers in children – "Come Ride the Magical Tunnel Of Love."

Capitellum – 2 years of age
Radial head – 4 years
Medial condyle – 6 years
Trochlea – 8 years
Olecrenon – 10 years
Lateral condyle – 12 years

98% of pediatric supracondylar distal humerus fx's are extension type (apex of fracture anterior).

Gartland Classification – Type I – non-displaced; Type II – anterior gapping with intact posterior hinge; Type III – no cortical continuity.

The conservative treatment for Gartland II/III is a trip to the OR for closed reduction and percutaneous pinning.

Reduction maneuver for extension type distal humerus fx's – full extension of elbow, align fx in varus/valgus plane, flex elbow and reduce anterior gapping by pressure on olecrenon, pronate wrist to lock fx in place.

<u>Pediatric Femur fx's</u>

Treatment:

Birth – 6 months – Pavlik harness or Spica cast.

6 months to 5 years – immediate spica if <2cm shortened, otherwise traction then spica cast.

6 years to 12 years – controversial – ex-fix/flexible IM rods/plating/immediate spica/traction, then spica all options.

>12 years – IM Nail – enter canal through the greater trochanter instead of piriformis fossa to reduce the risk of AVN.

<u>Tibial Spine fx's</u>

Meyers and McKeever classification:

Type I – minimal displacement
Type II – displaced but intact posterior hinge
Type III – complete separation of fragment with upward displacement and rotation

Treatment can be extension casting if an adequate reduction can be maintained; otherwise, treatment is ORIF.

Ankle fx's

Distal tibial physis closes asymmetrically (central first, then medial, finally lateral) starting about age 15. – This causes some unique adolescent ankle fx's.

Juvenile Tillaux fx– anterior inferior tibiofibular bony avulsion off tibia.

Triplane fx – slightly younger age than Tillaux fx-Salter-Harris II appearance on lateral X-ray; Salter-Harris III on A/P X-ray.

Shoulder/Humerus

SITS muscles – rotator cuff – In a right shoulder goes counter-clockwise from the top (Supraspinatus, Infraspinatus, Teres Minor, Subscapularis).

Triangular space – teres minor (superior), teres major (inferior), and long head of triceps (lateral) through which run circumflex scapular vessels.

Quadrangular space – teres minor (superior), teres major (inferior), long head of triceps (medial) and humerus (lateral) through which run the posterior humeral circumflex artery and axillary nerve.

Triangular interval – below Quad space – teres major (superior), long head triceps (medial) and lateral head of triceps (lateral) – The profunda brachii and radial nerve can be seen through this space, but they don't cross through it.

Proximal humerus fractures –

Neer classification separates proximal humerus into parts – greater tuberosity, lesser tuberosity.

Humeral head and shaft – If any part is separated from the others by 45 degrees of angulation or 1 cm, it is considered a separate part up to the maximum of four part fracture.

Check integrity of AXILLARY NERVE before manipulation of fracture by checking firing of deltoid muscle and sensation over "Sargeant's patch" of lateral arm.

Fracture Conference – Shoulder/Humerus

X-rays – A/P, lateral, axillary (can miss posterior dislocations without axillary view).

Treatment – reduction of any dislocation, followed by sling and swathe.

Many proximal humerus fractures can be treated non-operatively, save ORIF for physiologically younger, high demand patients. Hemi-arthroplasty for older patients with a four part or head splitting fracture.

As long as the shoulder is reduced, no need for immediate surgical intervention.

Surgical treatments include percutaneous pinning, ORIF, intramedullary nailing, and hemi-arthroplasty.

Humeral Shaft Fractures – "Put two ends of the humerus in the same room and they'll heal."—Marc Fuchs, M.D.

95% union rate with functional bracing (Sarmiento brace); in ER, initially put in a coaptation splint (medial and lateral plaster slats wrapped with Kerlex roll then ACE wrap). The fracture is usually unstable, and do not be surprised if it moves position several times over the first week to 10 days. If the patient is morbidly obese functional bracing may not work because the body habitus pushes the fracture into varus. Always check status of RADIAL NERVE by checking and documenting wrist/finger extension (Holstein-Lewis fractures-distal third spiral, oblique fractures-common for radial nerve to be out). If open fracture: plating or IM rod. If non-union: compression plating with bone graft.

Acromioclavicular (AC) joint dislocations –

Grade I – sprain of AC joint.
Grade II – partial displacement with AC ligament disruption.
Grade III – marked displacement with rupture of coracoclavicular ligaments.
Grade IV – complete dislocation with posterior displacement.
Grade V – >100% displacement superiorly with disruption of deltotrapezial fascia and sometimes skin tenting.
Grade VI – complete dislocation with inferior (subcoracoid) displacement.
Grade I and II – treat with sling; Grade IV-VI – surgery; Grade III – controversial (depends on age, occupation, and patient expectations).

Fracture Conference – Shoulder/Humerus, Spines

Seven things that attach to the coracoid-pectoralis minor, short head of biceps, coracobrachialis, coracohumeral ligament, coracoacromial ligament, and coracoclavicular ligaments (conoid-medial and trapezoid-lateral).

<u>Clavicle Fractures</u> –

The clavicle begins to ossify at 5 weeks in utero and the proximal clavicle ossification center does not fuse until age 22–25 years.

Group I – middle third; Group II – lateral; Group III – medial third.

Most clavicle fx's do well with conservative treatment (sling).

Indications for ORIF: open fx, neurovascular involvement, "floating shoulder" (ipsilateral clavicle/surgical neck of scapular fx), non-union of the clavicle.

Elective ORIF trades "a bump for a scar," i.e. don't operate for cosmesis alone.

Spine Fractures

C-spine – must have adequate lateral (from atlas to top of T1) – Ask for swimmer's view, repeat lateral or CT if cannot visualize. Most pathology is visible on lateral. All acute neuro out patients should be started on methylprednisolone, 30 mg/kg initial IV bolus and 23 hrs of 5.4 mg/kg IV.

Syndromes –

Central Cord – Most common, upper extremity affected more than lower extremities.

Brown-Sequard – Loss of ipsilateral motor function and contralateral pain and temperature sensation.
Posterior Cord – Extremely rare, preservation of motor fuction and loss of sensory function.
Anterior Cord – Less common, lower extremities affected more than upper, posterior column sensory pathways are spared.

In an adult on lateral film, anterior vertebral line, posterior vertebral line, spinolaminar line, and spinous processes should be smooth (no jump). Look closely at height of vertebral bodies and the disc spaces.

Fracture Conference – Spines, Open Fractures, Tumors

Lumbar spine – 3 column theory (anterior column – anterior 2/3 of body, anterior longitudinal ligament; middle column – posterior 1/3 of body, posterior longitudinal ligament; posterior column – facets, ligamentum flavum, spuraspinous ligament).

Compression fractures – most common-middle column remains intact-unstable if more than 50% loss of height or >30 degrees angulation.

Burst fractures – more severe-look for interpedicular widening on A/P – can have canal compromise (axial CT) – considered unstable if >50 loss of height or 50% spinal canal compromise – If stable, can treat with hyperextension bracing.

Chance fractures or "seat belt" fractures – mechanism is flexion/distraction – three column injury – anticipate visceral injury – if fracture is through the vertebral body ("Bony Chance fracture"), may heal with orthosis – if Chance injury through soft tissue, needs fusion.

Open Fractures

Gustilo and Anderson Classification:

Type I – clean wound <1 cm, minimal soft tissue injury.
Type II – wound >1 cm, moderate contamination, moderate soft tissue damage.
Type IIIA – wound>10 cm, high contamination.
Type IIIB – wound>10 cm, high contamination, severe soft tissue loss usually requiring a flap.
Type IIIC – wound>10 cm, high contamination, sever soft tissue loss plus vascular injury.

Antibiotics – Type I/II – Ancef 1gm IV q8 hr for 3 days.

Type III – Ancef plus Gentamycin 1.5 mg/kg q 8 hrs for 5 days.

Type III with barnyard, lake or stream contamination – add Penicillin 4 million units q6hrs for clostridium prophylaxis.

Tumors/Pathologic Fractures

Most common bone tumors are metastatic from PT Barnum Loves Kids-Prostrate, Thyroid, Breast, Lung, and Kidney.

Fracture Conference – Tumors

Metastatic Renal Cell Carcinoma is notoriously vascular-consider angiogram with embolization prior to surgery.

Also, think age for tumors:

Age	Common Tumors
0–3 years	Neuroblastoma, Rhabdomyosarcoma
3–10	Ewing's Sarcoma, Eosinopilic Granuloma
10–20	Osteosarcoma
20–50	Chondrosarcoma
>50	Malignant Fibrous Histiocytoma, Fibrosarcoma, Multiple Myeloma

Criteria for prophylactic internal fixation of impending fractures-painful, destructive lesion, 2.5 cm in diameter, loss of 50% or more of cortex of a long bone.

Common associated buzz words:

Vertebral plana (uniform compression of vertebrae in a child) – Eosinophilic Granuloma.

Sacral lesion or occipital tumor (destructive) and foamy, vaculoated cells ("physaliferous cells") – Chordoma.

Shepard's Crook (Varus proximal femur) – Fibrous Dysplasia.

Ewing's Sarcoma, Eosinophilic Granuloma, and infection – all three are always together in DDx.

Biphasic tumors (tumors with 2 cell types) – Adamantinoma, Synovial Sacroma, and Neurilemmoma.

Epiphyseal tumors – Chondroblastoma, Giant Cell Tumor, Clear Cell Chondrosarcoma.

"Corduroy Vertebae" (striation in vertebral body) or polka dot vertebral body on CT – Hemangioma .

"Erlenmeyer flask deformity" – Osteopetrosis.

Fracture Conference – Tumors, Nerves

Enneking Tumor Staging	Surgical resections
IA-Low grade, intracompartmental.	Intralesional-biopsy through the lesion.
IB-Low grade, extracompartmental.	Marginal-resection through the reactive zone.
IIA-High grade, intracompartmental.	Wide-entire tumor with reactive zone removed.
IIB-High grade, extracompartmental.	Radical-entire tumor with its associated compartment. removed.

IIIA-intracompartmental with metastasis

IIIB-extracompartmental with metastasis

Motor Exam

Nerve root	Muscles	Reflex
C4	Scapular musculature	None
C5	Deltoid, biceps	Biceps
C6	Biceps, wrist extensors, triceps	Brachioradialis
C7	Triceps, wrist flexors	Triceps
C8	Finger flexors, interossei	None
T1	Interossei	None
L2, L3	Iliopsoas (hip flexors)	None
L4	Quadriceps, tibialis anterior	Patellar
L5	EHL	None
S1	Gastroc/soleus complex	Achilles
S2–S4	Bowel/bladder	Cremasteric

CERVICAL AND THORACIC DERMATOMES

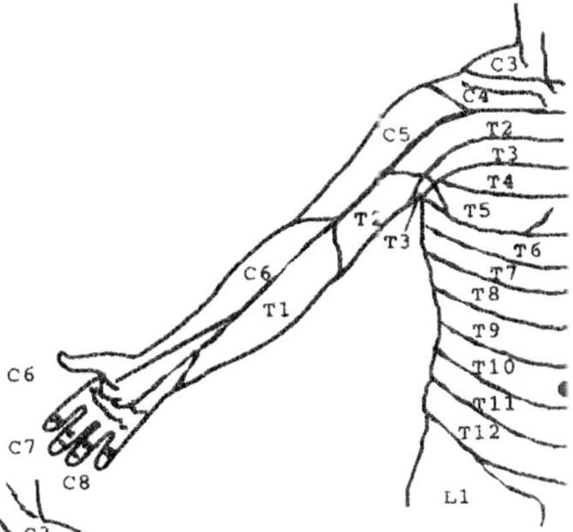

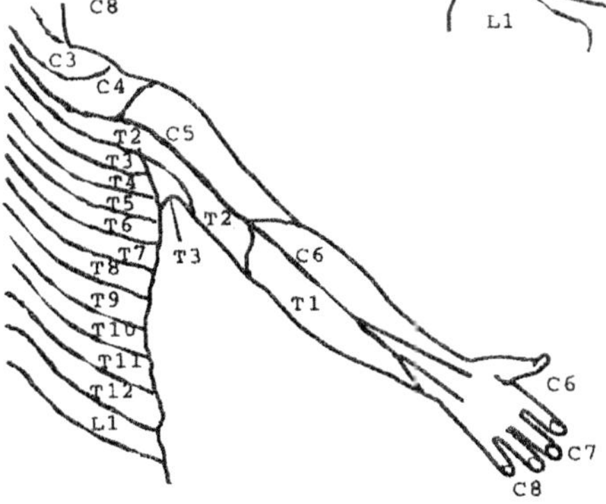

LOWER THORACIC AND LUMBOSACRAL DERMATOMES

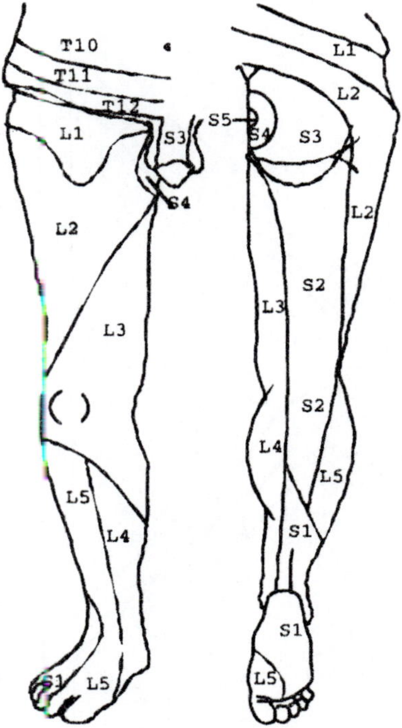

BRACHIAL PLEXUS

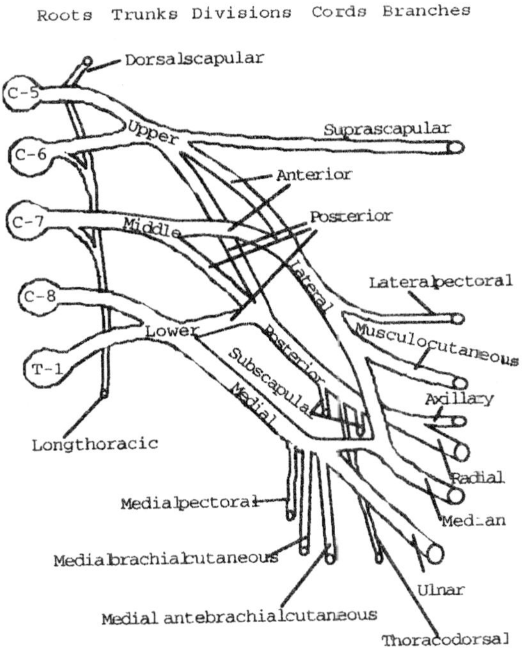

MEDIAN NERVE

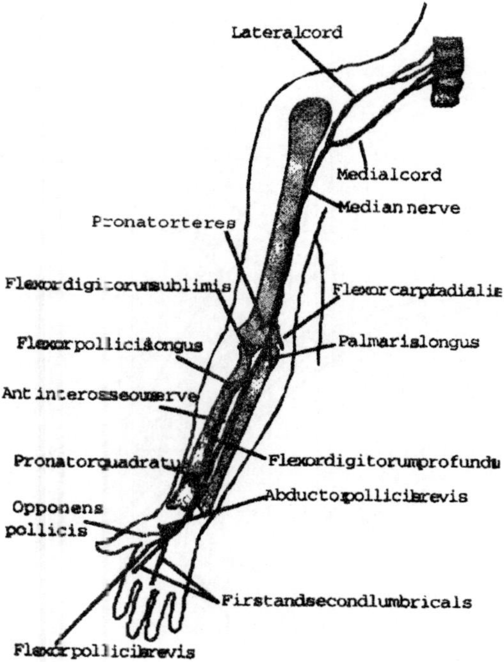

RADIAL NERVE

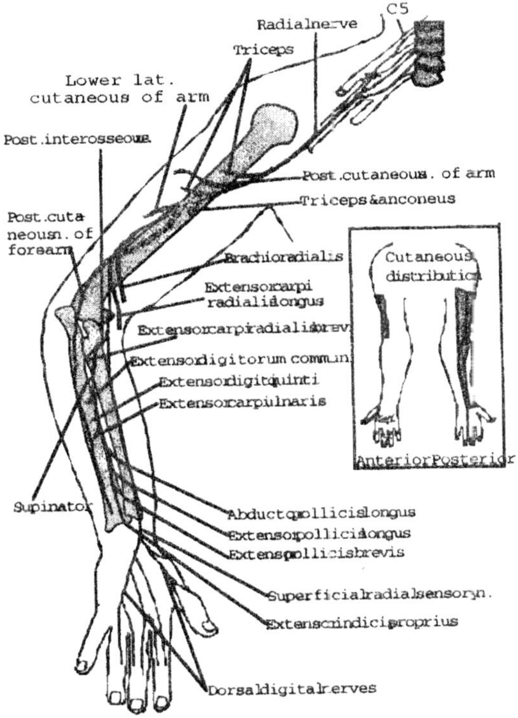

ULNAR NERVE

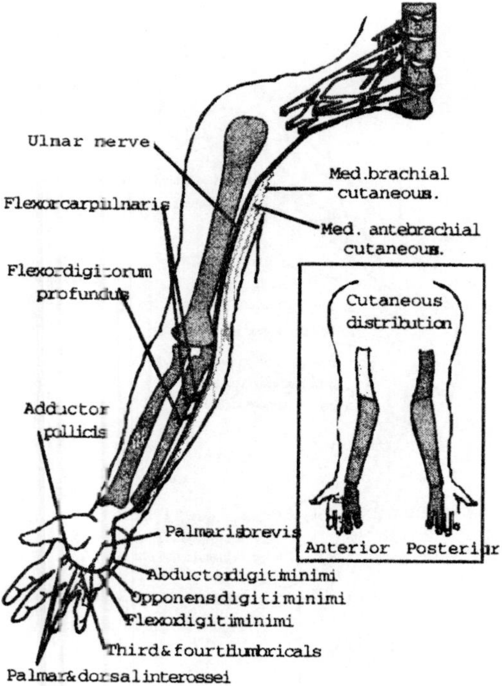

Ulnar nerve
Med.brachial cutaneous.
Flexorcarpiulnaris
Med. antebrachial cutaneous.
Flexordigitorum profundus
Cutaneous distribution
Adductor pollicis
Palmarisbrevis
Anterior
Posterior
Abductordigitiminimi
Opponensdigitiminimi
Flexordigitiminimi
Third& fourthlumbricals
Palmar& dorsalinterossei

SCIATIC NERVE

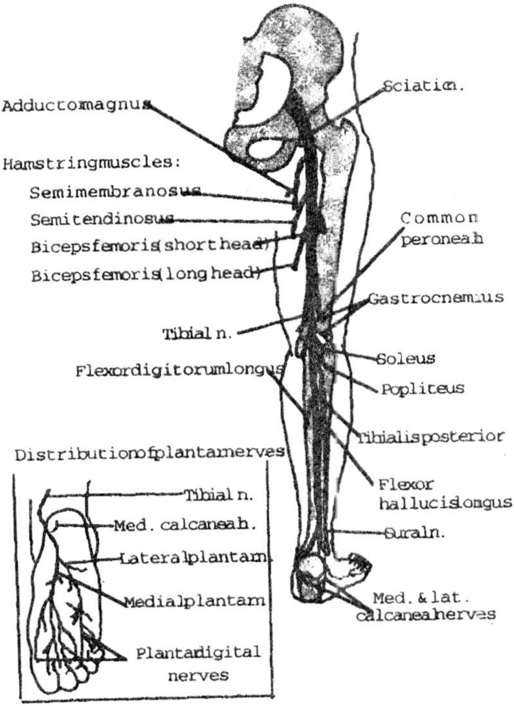

Lumbosacral Plexus

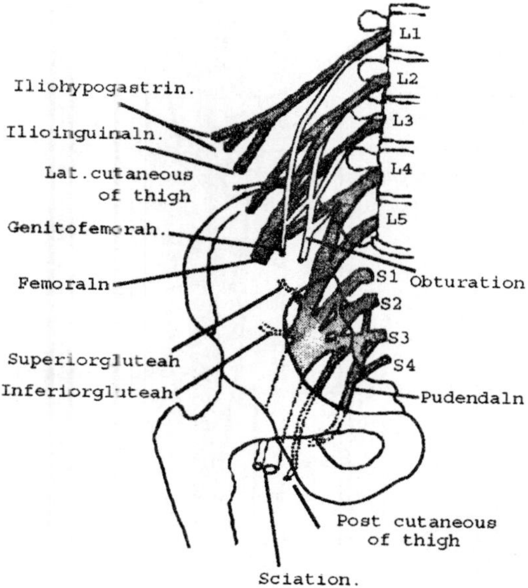

Suggested Reading List

Your time is valuable. Here's a list of books that are worth spending that time.

1. *Hoppenfeld's Physical Exam of the Spine and Extremities* -Your job is getting a history and physical and then reporting your findings, and understanding the techniques in this thin book is a great start.
2. *Rockwood and Green's Fractures in Adults and Children*-I read this cover to cover as an intern, which helped me throughout my residency. It gives you a solid understanding of fractures and their treatment and is a great reference source. The historical reviews can drag on, so skim them unless you get jazzed about learning which historical figures died from a clavicle fracture (by the way, it's Sir Robert Peel and William III).
3. *Skeletal Trauma*-More to the point than Rockwood and Green. Also a great reference source for all fractures.
4. *Hoppenfeld's Surgical Exposures*-Hard to believe that most surgeries you do as an orthopaedic surgeon rely on the approaches in this one inch book, but it's true. Also great anatomy review.
5. *OKU*-Summarizes the latest advances and current treatments for many orthopaedic conditions. It is <u>not</u> a comprehensive textbook for all disorders.
6. *Miller's Review of Orthopaedics*-Great for OITE review. Its outline format gives you a good sampling about almost all orthopaedic conditions, but reading it as a primary source will leave gaps in your knowledge. Use the excellent bibliography at the end of each chapter.
7. *Orthopaedic Basic Science*-The OITE and the Boards are stressing basic science more and more. Drink plenty of coffee before tackling this book.
8. *Journal of the American Academy of Orthopaedic Surgeons*-The "Yellow Journal." All excellent review articles that are a great way to be introduced to advanced topics, 7–8 at a time.

Notes

Notes

International Medical Publishing, Inc.

Intern Pocket Survival Guides

the Intern Pocket Survival Guide $ 9.50
the CCU Intern Pocket Survival Guide $ 9.50
the ER Intern Pocket Survival Guide $ 9.50
the ICU Intern Pocket Survival Guide $ 9.50
the Surgical Intern Pocket Survival Guide $ 9.50
the Oncology Intern Pocket Survival Guide $ 9.50

the Gastroenterology Resident Pocket Survival Guide $9.95

Emergency Handbooks

the EKG Pocket Survival Guide $ 7.50
the ACLS Pocket Survival Guide $ 7.50

Order Form

In addition to your address, please include an e-mail or phone number so that we might contact you with any questions about your order.

Name: ______________________________

Address: ______________________________

City, State, Zip: ______________________________

Daytime phone/e-mail: ______________________________

Please send a Personal Check or Credit Card (circle one):

Visa Mastercard

Card Number ______________________ Expiration ________

Signature ______________________________

Title		Quantity	Price
	Tax 5% VA		
	S&H		$5.95
	Total		

Sale Tax 5% VA
Shipping charges are $5.95 for first book and 50 cents each additional
Please call for other rates.
Please send your order to:

International Medical Publishing, Inc.
PO Box 479
McLean, VA 22101

Information and ordering: 800-530-3142 Fax: (703) 7348987
E-mail inquiries to: orders@medicalpublishing.com.
online: www.medicalpublishing.com

Notes